Communication

Active Listening, And Public Speaking Improved And
Social Intelligence

*(Effective Strategies For Enhancing Communication And
Strengthening Relationships)*

Basil Hodgkinson

TABLE OF CONTENT

Introduction

Public speaking is communicating to a group of people in a structured, deliberate manner with the intention of informing, persuading, or entertaining the audience. It is a form of communication in which the speaker addresses an audience and conveys a message through vocal techniques and body language.

Public speaking is an essential skill that is applicable in a variety of contexts, including academic, professional, and personal circumstances. It enables speakers to effectively communicate their ideas and thoughts to a large audience and can be used to educate, inform, inspire, or persuade the audience.

There are many advantages to acquiring public speaking skills. It can help individuals develop self-assurance and poise, enhance their ability to think on their feet and communicate effectively, and strengthen their leadership abilities. As the ability to communicate effectively is highly valued in many professions, public speaking can also help people advance their careers. In addition, public speaking can be a potent instrument for social change because it enables individuals to raise awareness about significant issues and advocate for causes they believe in.

When delivering a public speech or presentation, it is common for people to feel nervous or anxious. This is commonly referred to as performance anxiety or stage nervousness. Up to 75% of individuals experience some degree of stage fright when speaking in public, according to research.

Lack of confidence in one's speaking abilities, dread of failure or negative evaluation, and unfamiliarity with the audience or subject matter are all potential causes of stage fright. Some individuals may also experience physical symptoms of stage anxiety, such as an elevated heart rate, profuse sweating, and trembling.

Even though stage fright is a normal and prevalent experience, it is manageable and can be overcome with preparation and practice. Numerous individuals find it beneficial to familiarize themselves with their material, rehearse their delivery, and employ techniques such as deep breathing and visualization to calm their nerves. Obtaining support from friends, coworkers, or a professional therapist can also aid in overcoming stage anxiety.

There are numerous benefits associated with overcoming stage anxiety and becoming a fearless speaker. Among the prospective advantages of overcoming stage fright are:

Public speaking can be intimidating, but through practice and preparation, individuals can increase their confidence and become more at ease when speaking in front of others.

Communication skills can be improved through practice and overcoming stage anxiety. Public speaking requires clear and effective communication, which can be improved through practice.

The ability to speak in front of a group with assurance can help individuals establish themselves as leaders and inspire others to follow their ideas.

The ability to speak in public with confidence is highly valued in many professions, and overcoming stage fright can lead to new job opportunities or promotions.

Influence: The ability to communicate persuasively and with self-assurance enables individuals to advocate for causes they care about and have a positive impact on their communities.

Overcoming stage anxiety and becoming a fearless speaker can help individuals develop self-assurance, enhance their communication skills, and boost their leadership and career prospects.

Chapter 1: Figure Out How To Appreciate Your Children In Public.

This is how to acknowledge your child's efforts and achievements and keep them energized!

In any case, would it be prudent for you to generally avoid praise? No, you only need to meticulously direct it. Careful recognition can be an extraordinary addition to your collection of nurturing tools. Therefore, the next time you wish to laud your child, try substituting the following expressions for your usual ones.

Here are 10 examples of effective recognition proclamations to try with your child:

Rather than saying "Well done!"

Attempt: "I appreciate your assistance with the cleanup. I particularly admire the manner in which the shoes have been arranged. This will have a significant impact on our efforts to locate our shoes at the beginning of the day.

One of the keys to more potent applause is being explicit. "Great job" is imprecise because it does not specify what the child did to earn your praise, it does not provide constructive criticism, and it does not indicate what behavior they should adopt in the future.

Related: why you should really praise yourself in front of your children, mother

Specify precisely what you are happy about. Mention why it satisfied you, with the hope that they will repeat it in the future. Specifically, explicitness helps them to feel respected.

Rather than saying "You did it!"

"I have observed you attempting to secure your shoelaces for quite some time. It's hazardous, right? Nevertheless, I am delighted that you persisted and did not give up. I'm confident that you'll get it shortly with your training and perseverance!"

Acknowledge the effort, not the outcome. Rapidly demoralize and demotivate a child by focusing solely on accomplishments. It is acceptable to commend achievement, but it is more important to commend the work that preceded that achievement. Applauding effort convinces and demonstrates confidence in the child.

Instead of "You look so attractive/pretty!"

Try: "I adore the creatures on your T-shirt; which is your favorite? Why is that the case?

Adulating children, especially young women, for their appearance can diminish their confidence. They may begin to believe that people like them solely because of their appearance, which can lead to a tremendous amount of tension as they age.

Appropriating a child's appearance can unintentionally associate their identity with their appearance. To compliment a child's appearance, emphasize what the child can alter. For instance, use the child's clothing to spark a conversation that demonstrates your genuine interest in what they think and feel.

Instead of, "That is an extraordinary drawing!"

Attempt: "Wow, I adore the variety you've chosen for the flowers; why did you decide to paint them in that color?"

This year, you may have viewed a hundred works of art, but to your child, each is extraordinary and new. Despite the fact that it may be simpler to state, "This is an excellent drawing" without actually examining it, what matters most to children is that they examine the artwork properly.

Choosing portions of the image and requesting information about their decisions demonstrates that you are genuinely interested in and appreciative of their work. Which, in child parlance, translates to you noticing and valuing them.

5. Instead of "Method for going, mate!"

Attempt: "You really exerted so much effort on that piece of work. I am pleased that your instructor has recognized this. You deserve that grade. Is there anything you've learned from this article that you can later apply to your own work?"

Observe your child's behavior if he or she focuses. Let them know you observed their sincere effort and that their work was valued. When they receive a passing grade, instead of merely praising the result, discuss with them what went well. This is an exceptional opportunity to help future school by requiring the student to consider the cycles and activities that led to the passing grade and to implement them again in the future.

Instead of "Outstanding young lady!"

"You worked diligently on that numerical question. I recognize you could address it if you were genuinely interested!"

Commending children for fixed credits, such as intelligence or aptitude in specific subjects, can backfire. Not only will children avoid making a solid effort in the future if they believe they are naturally good at something, but they will also become promptly frustrated if they encounter difficulty, assuming they are intelligent all things considered.

Chapter 2: How To Make Your Introduction

Cold tremors, perspiring palms, a trembling voice, a parched mouth, and eyes that do not know where to gaze. Hands that are incapable of proper behavior. Or it is not as terrible as it seems. You may have a well-rehearsed vocabulary of frequently used words. But can you introduce yourself in a way that will leave a lasting impression?

Introductions are inevitable. There are numerous motivations to do it. Perhaps a job interview or a complete stranger on a plane. Or perhaps at a social event or convention. A well-written and effective self-introduction can help you secure a job, close a business deal, and make new friends.

However, this requires some talent. Like a potter at his wheel, we must create something we can present with pride to others and, in doing so, leave an indelible and enduring impression.

A strong introduction will distinguish you from the rest of the crowd. Also, it will connect. Solve obstacles. And provide some satisfaction. Be intelligent and not too modest.

Conflict Resolution Methodology

Now that you are aware of your limits and what you are willing to tolerate, it is simpler to find a solution to a conflict. You can use a formula to guide you through the process while adapting the principles to the nature of the conflict.

Step 1: Determine the Conflict's Root Cause

This requires investigating the available information regarding the conflict's root cause. This will help you discover a solution that is unique to your situation, and it can be accomplished by asking questions.

What sequence of events led up to the incident?

When did you become aware that you were uneasy?

How long has this been taking place?

What is the connection between this incident and other occurrences?

Everyone involved must be able to convey themselves without prejudice. Not only will it provide them with the opportunity to debrief, but it will also provide you with the chance to gather information from everyone and make better decisions.

What is the larger perspective?

Frequently, you will receive a biased account of an incident, which can exacerbate tensions within the group. It is in everyone's best interest to determine the source of the tension so that the issue can be resolved and team members do not attack one another.

Step 3: Ask for Solutions

Inquire of your team members how they believe the situation can be resolved, asking them reflective questions about their relationship with one another and how their tension affected the remainder of the team. Keep the conversation focused on the current topic, and avoid asking queries that could lead to a blame game.

Find a solution that works for everyone

Consider several options that could result in a solution to the problem that benefits everyone. Collaboration will increase the positive outcomes of the organization and improve the performance of the team.

Fifth step: concurrence

The team must concur with what has been discussed. Especially if their personalities are incompatible and harmony is not guaranteed, it may be beneficial to have a contract drawn up to bind them to the agreement. The following inquiries can aid the situation:

How can future conflicts be prevented?

What will you do if an analogous circumstance occurs?

What are the repercussions if one of the parties violates the contract?

Chapter 3: How To Become A Compassionate Listener And Conversationalist

The skill of observing is a valuable asset. Understanding someone's perspective and gaining insight into their message can be beneficial. When people are intent on passing judgment, they frequently overlook the point the speaker is attempting to make. The art of listening necessitates genuine interest in what others have to say, regardless of whether you agree with them or would prefer they say something else. We form opinions because we believe we can perform better than others. The skill of listening enables you to be receptive to an alternative viewpoint, which you may find unexpected or even enlightening.

8. Provide feed-back

The art of effective communication is merely the ability to hear not only what a person says but also what they say. Do not be hesitant to express your thoughts on what the other person has said. If it is positive, give them a compliment. If it is negative, inform them. If a person informs you that they cannot receive information from another individual in a particular format, let them know; this will enable you to find solutions to this problem and possibly prevent it from occurring.

Communication is an extremely potent tool. It can provide us with extraordinary opportunities and adventures. Communication is bidirectional; whatever you send into the universe, whether positive or negative, will always return to you. The same applies to communication; if you want others to trust you and feel secure sharing their problems and life experiences with you, you must reciprocate when they open up to you. If we send out specific signals or indications that we are unwilling to heed, people will shut down communication with us. This means they will cease sharing their thoughts and emotions with us because they do not trust us to listen without judging or interfering. Being a good listener is not always simple, but it can be one of the most rewarding skills you ever acquire. Listening more will make all the difference in your relationships, so don't squander the opportunity.

Being an empathetic observer involves focusing on the other person's intent and message. It involves being deferential in your speech, tone, and facial expressions. It also involves focusing on the individual's requirements, wants, desires, and objectives. A good listener is receptive to what others have to say, asks pertinent questions when necessary, and expresses interest in hearing what they have to say. They will feel valued and embraced by the other individual. Being an empathetic listener requires more than just words; it also requires demonstrating personal and professional concern for others.

Being an effective listener requires time and effort. It is not something that can be completed readily overnight. The discipline of listening entails not only hearing another person's words, but also understanding their intention. Good listeners will take the time necessary to comprehend what the other person is saying. They ensure they fully comprehend the message, regardless of how challenging or unsettling it may initially appear. It does not matter how long it takes to completely comprehend what someone is saying; they will do whatever is necessary to grasp the message.

To be an empathetic listener, one must prioritize the other individual. It makes no difference what the other person says or how they express it. It only matters that their requirements and wants are satisfied. Their emotions are more essential than yours; it doesn't matter what you want as long as you can help them achieve their goals. The art of listening requires a willingness to embrace others for who they are, flaws and all, without judging who they ought to be or ought to have been.

A excellent listener is nonjudgmental and receptive to all communication from others. They avoid jumping to conclusions and strive to maintain composure when communicating. They do not evaluate the content or delivery of others' speech. They accept the sentiments and thoughts of others without becoming defensive or offended. A good listener is curious about what another person has to say, who they are, and their ambitions, dreams, aspirations, and objectives.

Patience and an appreciation of human nature are essential components of the art of listening. It takes time to cultivate good listening skills. The discipline of listening requires undivided attention to the person with whom one is conversing. It involves understanding how their mind functions, absorbing what they have just said, and recognizing all the emotions that may be guiding their actions and expressions. It also involves the ability to hear implicit messages in addition to spoken ones.

Chapter 4: Format For Enhancing Communication Abilities

Spend some time observing and recording your interactions with the people around you. Examine your speaking style, focusing on diction, volume, and tone. Examine your writing approach with a focus on language, syntax, and organization.

Recognize any problems, contradictions, or defects in your interpersonal interactions. Your strategy for development will center on these problem areas.

Determine the circumstances in which you are most and least comfortable implementing change.

Adjust your current objectives to accommodate newly discovered short-term objectives.

5. Look for opportunities to "practice" and keep an eye out for feedback opportunities along the way. Self-evaluation and self-monitoring are also advantageous when evaluating your development.

It is essential to exercise perseverance throughout the process, as self-improvement of any kind can be lengthy. There are available support programs and templates for anyone who believes they require assistance with any of the processes listed above. Numerous academic institutions, as well as qualified counselors and tutors, offer courses and seminars that teach communication skills to participants. Similarly, a person can evaluate their skills and limitations in communication by completing a variety of online tests.

After deciding to improve one's communication skills, there are a few straightforward suggestions that can aid in this enlightening process:

- When speaking, remember to speak at a slow, appropriate pace, to pause when necessary, and to endeavor to pronounce your words clearly in order to avoid slurring.

- When speaking, focus on using the appropriate volume, including volume adjustments for emphasis when necessary, and the appropriate tone.

- Prepare for events such as gatherings and public speaking engagements. Take the time to review names and backgrounds in advance if you frequently experience breakdowns or protracted pauses in these situations.

Practice posing queries to yourself and answering them. For instance, you might inquire, "How have you been?" Then, you should inquire, "What have you been doing?" Recognize the context of the engagement: a formal event requires a different communication style than an informal one, necessitating a different application of these skills.

At any stage in their lives, anyone can benefit from effective communication skills. These soft skills are crucial for a joyful, long-lasting family life and are in high demand in the business world.Improving your communication skills may have a significant impact on numerous aspects of your existence. You can anticipate an increase in your enjoyment, self-assurance, and social success.

Throughout the process of enhancing communication, the elimination of communication barriers is crucial. People frequently develop barriers and anxieties due to previous communication failures, and it can be difficult to overcome these obstacles. Due to a lack of confidence, a person might speak rapidly or avoid eye contact while listening. They could avoid interacting with strangers and fighting with family members or coworkers. You can convey your thoughts and emotions more effectively if you improve your communication skills. These enhancements are applicable everywhere, including the bedroom and the boardroom.

When asked what effective communication skills mean to them, the average person frequently overlooks the importance of listening. To successfully communicate, one must be a confident and proactive listener. Both listening and communicating are essential to effective communication. Understanding the person or people with whom you are interacting and establishing a stronger rapport with them are dependent on attentive listening. A person's ability to empathize and sympathize with others is enhanced by their skillful expression of sadness, pleasure, or regret.

By enhancing their communication skills, the individual significantly enhances their possibilities for personal development. Strong communication skills can significantly improve a leader's ability to inspire coworkers and family members. Effective communication skills are essential for managing personal tension from the perspective of self-maintenance. A person can become more assertive by enhancing the effectiveness of his or her communication, which includes the ability to take charge of a discussion or situation and achieve the desired result. Better communication skills can considerably increase a person's capacity to manage conflicts at home and at work.

The ability to communicate effectively enables one to carry oneself with greater self-assurance and present a dynamic and sociable attitude, which increases one's likelihood of finding love or making new acquaintances. These enhancements to a person's personal development will also improve their networking skills. Effective networking is a crucial success factor in today's global, competitive job market, and this reality is only growing. The ability to "schmooze" with top management or endear oneself to business executives may lead to an increase in responsibility, pay, and career opportunities.

Physical communication is crucial for effective communication and includes fidgeting, hand gestures, and eye movements. Additionally, many believe that it is the most challenging aspect to monitor and improve. People frequently pay such close attention to what they are saying or hearing that they fail to notice how they are moving.

It is difficult for the average person to acquire the skill of public speaking. Maintaining the audience's interest while conveying a crucial message requires skill. A successful communicator may find a way to bring their speech to life and use both their voice and physical presence to captivate and inform their audience.

Understanding the person or group with whom you are communicating is essential for effective communication. A proficient communicator must distinguish between appropriate and inappropriate humor and decorum. Even though it has the potential to be a powerful ally, humor can quickly turn against you if it is used haphazardly and without discretion.

Effective written language usage is a crucial component of effective communication skills. Despite their education and degrees, a large number of people find that their writing skills are deficient. As with many aspects of life, the development of writing skills must be addressed progressively and through the use of trainer signals. A fast "loves" and "dislikes" list or even a small apology to someone is a good idea. Effective writing requires the use of plain, emotive language to make a point while avoiding "offending" the reader's sensibilities with unnecessary jargon.

Chapter 5: Obstacles To Successful Workplace Communication

Numerous individuals typically characterize the workplace as tense, hectic, productive, and perhaps even a source of distraction for others. Without straightforward communication, many things are misunderstood, and managers frequently make poor decisions due to a lack of clarity. Establishing a profit is the primary purpose for establishing a business. Why would a corporation risk their reputation and continued existence due to poor communication?

There are obstacles to effective workplace communication. In order to foster productive communication, both managers and employees must be aware of these obstacles and take the necessary steps to eliminate them. Why is this important? The most embarrassing thing you can do is base a business decision on what you believe you heard or comprehended.

Distractions

When managers meet in a boardroom or cubicle, they share the information necessary for making business decisions. Managers should consider conducting meetings in a location with few interruptions. Cellphones are an undeniable distraction in boardrooms, especially when personalized ringtones interrupt essential information-sharing discussions. If managers rely solely on what they believe to have heard without obtaining clarification, they run the risk of making a poor business decision. Distractions can take a variety of forms. Holding a meeting in an environment where participants cannot hear what is being said is a recipe for disaster.

Stress

While some employees flourish under stress, others may find it difficult to manage it at work. When firms are thriving or struggling, managers and employees frequently act hastily or without complete information. You can better manage your tension by learning to prioritize events and their relative importance (as they occur).

Attitudes

This is an important issue because an individual's attitude can severely hinder communication. This mentality could be held by either management or workers. When attitudes are accounted for, emotions will enter the equation. Everyone desires to be correct; everyone desires to accuse others of being incorrect, and everyone desires to be correct. When it comes to establishing the tone for the communication process, both management and each individual have a professional obligation to take a firm stance.

Language

Tone, intonation, and popular phrases are interpreted differently by individuals, particularly when they speak a foreign language. You must be cognizant of this, English-speaking managers and employees. This is indicative of the reality of a diverse workplace. It is irresponsible to express irritation with a colleague who has a strong accent. Diversity in the workplace will never cease to exist.

Last but not least, the company's internal structure is frequently a barrier to effective communication. When employees are required to adhere to organizational charts, communication between supervisors and upper management is often impeded. I believe that the value of effective workplace communication is realized when managers and supervisors are able to receive timely and useful feedback from senior management in order to make prudent business decisions.

Chapter 6: The Real Keys To Effective Communication

You can learn to communicate effectively and efficiently with others through a variety of techniques. You can finish each exercise, beginning with A. Even if you perfect your vocal pitch, say what you mean and mean what you say, and move your body appropriately, there will always be something missing.

Some things merely demand our attention, whereas others have the exact opposite effect. Do you appreciate conversing with uninteresting and self-centered individuals? What are your thoughts on conversing with someone who does not appear to be listening? How do you feel when you have a wonderful, two-way conversation with someone who is beaming from ear to ear and anxious to hear what you have to say? There are tremendous disparities.

You will be able to communicate with anyone, anywhere, and accomplish your goals if you go above and beyond. You are not a wall, so conversing with you will not be like talking to a wall. Genuine communication is always worth the additional effort required for its success. It's like the icing on the cake. Now let's begin preparing!

I Want What He Has: A Technique for Achieving His Smile

You have undoubtedly heard of "How to Win Friends and Influence People," Dale Carnegie's infamous 1936 self-improvement book. According to an old proverb, your smile conveys your good will. Perhaps you've even read the book. Everyone who sees your smile feels better. Someone who has observed a dozen people grimace, frown, or turn their features away will find your smile to be like the sun breaking through the clouds.

While Mr. Carnegie's observations are accurate, a smile does not always ensure acceptance and a sympathetic ear. The author Leil Lowndes explains in his book "How to Talk to Anyone: 92 Little Tricks for Big Success in Relationships" that a smile may be the key to communication, or it may prevent it.

Everyone has encountered a salesperson with a forced expression. Because it is expected of him, he beams. He is intent on a solitary concept. He desires to gain profit from you. This type of expression is certainly repulsive.

Conversely, some individuals have a smile that extends like a yawn. When someone grins at you, you reflexively smile back. These individuals are uplifting and encourage you to attend to them. You are intrigued by their point of view. You covet what they have.

Mr. Carnegie is, all things considered, unquestionably accurate. Also, Leil

Lowndes is. Unquestionably, the ideal smile can transform you into a conversing machine. The improper smirk, such as a forced or sarcastic one, may immediately repel people. In order for your smile to be effective and not work against you, it must be flawless. In fact, I'm devoting a substantial amount of material to it due to its importance. Ready?

the importance of beaming. A smile is as bright as the sun. As parents, we are ecstatic because it is one of the first methods in which infants learn to communicate. While infants wail from birth, the first time they smile is a developmental milestone. In addition to communicating their requirements and desires, they are also communicating their emotions. A infant will smile when they are content. There is nothing sweeter than this. When we are pleased, we smile, and seeing others smile often makes us smile as well.

The science behind a grin. In an article titled "Untapped Power of Smiling" on Forbes.com, Ron Gutman explains the principles behind smiling.

In his article, Gutman concluded, "Smiling stimulates our brain's reward circuits in a way that even chocolate, a sluggish pleasure inducer, cannot match."

What exactly occurs in the brain during a smile that is so extraordinary that it may be superior to unadulterated chocolate? Let's get to it: Something favorable occurs. A neuronal signal travels from the cortex of the brain to the medulla, where it is processed by the cranial muscles before reaching the muscles that cause you to smile. Nevertheless, there's more! After you smile, your brain receives a positive feedback loop, which causes you to feel joyful. Wow! That is something to celebrate!

Dial with a smile. I was a telemarketer in the past, although I'm not precisely bragging about it. I am, indeed, the person you hung up on. It is also conceivable that I am one of the few telemarketers with whom you have interacted. Why? My supervisor positioned a mirror at each of our workstations. It was our obligation to smile. We were instructed to smile while dressing and during every phone call. Considering that the person on the other end of the line couldn't even see me, you may question what purpose that served. Surprisingly, it is possible to hear individuals smiling while they are speaking. Try it. You will make the decision. I can absolutely attest to that. Regardless of whether the individual or people you are speaking with can see you or not, you will receive entirely different responses when you smile versus when you do not.

Make things up along the way? Surely you've heard the adage, "Fake it until you make it." Does this, however, extend to a smile? Even though this occurs on occasion, recall the salesperson. A fake smile may be interpreted as deceit, ridicule, or another negative emotion. Attempting to fake a smile in order to make yourself and others pleased is a very different situation. Once we examine the various types of smiles, you'll have a greater understanding of their differences.

power game Smiles are infectious. It is the ideal method for spreading pleasure and influencing the happiness of others. Nothing is more effective in verbal communication for gaining attention. People are receptive. They will compete for what you have.

Chapter 7: Realize The Importance Of Self-Confidence

Successful negotiators share a common trait of self-assurance. They always appear in charge of themselves and their negotiation contacts. How can you attain this aura of confidence? Before meeting with your adversaries, thoroughly consider your alternatives to settlement. Once you comprehend your options, you will no longer feel fear. Your self-assurance is likely to influence your fellow negotiators. If your competitors perceive that their non-settlement options are less appealing than the options available to you, they will be under greater pressure to negotiate. This is when they begin to make greater and greater concessions.

When your self-confidence begins to wane, which happens to even the most self-confident among us, and you begin to doubt your negotiating skills, you should do two things:

Consider the weaknesses of your opponents so that you can exploit what they are concealing. They are highlighting their strengths, and you must predict what flaws they are concealing.

2. reevaluate your own circumstance to determine which of your strengths you are showcasing. If you do a good job of concealing your own weaknesses, your competitors may presume you have greater strength than you actually do. Reconsider your non-settlement options and concentrate on the alternatives available to your opponents. Avoid giving your opponent false strength.

When I serve as a negotiator's consultant for attorneys, they do a fantastic job of highlighting their own side's defects. When I put myself in their opponents' shoes and explain the challenges they confront, the attorneys with whom I work are stunned. They have completely ignored the obstacles that their opponents confront. At this time, they begin to recognize their negotiating strength.

When making concessions, adhere to your principles. Position adjustments must be strategically planned and communicated. When used appropriately, a concession can convey both a cooperative attitude and sufficient firmness to imply the need for a counteroffer if the negotiator wishes to continue the negotiation process. Intelligent negotiators begin the distributive phase with principled positions that logically justify their desires. Make principled concessions that you can adequately defend to your competitors. When placing a new position on the table, provide an explanation for your decision. You can argue that you undervalued or overvalued a particular item by a certain amount, and then modify your current position accordingly. You may also assert that you neglected to conduct a thorough analysis of a crucial piece of information and subsequently modify your current offer accordingly. This strategy causes you to halt at your opponent's new position, as opposed to a higher or lower one, and causes them to question whether their own positions are still valid or need to be revised.

When a person surrenders unexpectedly, it indicates anxiety and a lack of self-control. This especially true when a position shift is made tentatively and without integrity by an individual who continues to speak awkwardly and defensively after the compromise. This action demonstrates a lack of confidence and informs the other party that the individual who has just shifted roles does not expect immediate reciprocity. When you encounter such concession-makers, gently encourage them to continue conversing, as their approach frequently results in additional concessions that go unanswered. If you can induce competitors to bid against themselves through successive position changes, you should be able to seize control of the interaction and generate favorable results. If none is forthcoming immediately, wait patiently for the recipient to resume the conversation. This notifies him or her that you will not take any further action until his or her initial move is reciprocated.

Chapter 8: Different contexts for communication

Workplace communication

Effective communication at work is necessary for establishing and sustaining positive relationships with coworkers, effectively resolving problems, and achieving organizational objectives. Here are some communication guidelines for the workplace:

Listen carefully: Attend to what others are saying and demonstrate that you are participating in the conversation. Avoid interrupting or multitasking.

Use clear and concise language: Be clear and concise in your communication, and avoid jargon or technical terms that may not be understood by all.

Use a businesslike tone: Communicate in a professional manner and avoid using vernacular or inappropriate language.

Consider your audience: Consider the recipient of your message and adjust it accordingly. This can enable you to communicate more effectively.

Be respectful: Respect others and their ideas, and refrain from employing censure or criticism.

Effectively communicate in writing by using correct grammar and spelling, as well as being plain and concise.

Effective communication at work requires active listening, the use of plain and concise language, a professional tone, consideration of the audience, respect, and effective written communication. By implementing these suggestions, you can enhance your communication skills and navigate the workplace more effectively.

interacting in social settings

Effective communication in social situations is essential for establishing and sustaining relationships and fostering a positive social experience. Here are some communication guidelines for social situations:

Listen carefully: Attend to what others are saying and demonstrate that you are participating in the conversation. Avoid interrupting or multitasking.

Use open-ended questions: Asking open-ended inquiries can aid in gaining a deeper understanding of others and promote discussion and dialogue.

Be respectful: Respect others and their ideas, and refrain from employing censure or criticism.

Use nonverbal cues: Employ nonverbal cues such as eye contact, facial expressions, and body language to demonstrate interest in the conversation.

Consider the feelings and requirements of others, and make an effort to be understanding and empathetic.

Use excellent manners, such as saying "please" and "thank you," to demonstrate respect and courtesy.

Effective communication in social situations requires active listening, the use of open-ended questions, respect, the use of nonverbal cues, consideration for others, and excellent manners. By adhering to these guidelines, you can enhance your communication skills and create a more enjoyable social experience.

Chapter 9: Conflict Resolution Through Negotiation And Compromise

Good parenting requires the ability to compromise and negotiate, as disagreements are a natural part of parenthood. When conflicts arise, parents must approach the situation with composure, an open mind, and a willingness to listen to their child. By negotiating and compromising with their children, parents can assist their children in developing critical problem-solving skills and a deeper, more affectionate bond.

Establishing norms and limits with a child can serve as an example of how to use negotiation and compromise to solve a problem.

As they strive for autonomy, children have a natural inclination to question societal norms and limitations. Rather than imposing rules without the child's input, parents may negotiate a set of rules that is acceptable to both the parent and the child. Throughout this process, the child may communicate their desires and requirements, and the parent may share their concerns and justifications. Using this method, both parties may arrive at a solution that takes into account the requirements and perspectives of the parent and the child.

When establishing boundaries and rules with a child, for instance, compromise and negotiation can be beneficial. A parent could, for instance, designate a time for their child to return home from school on weeknights so that they have sufficient rest before class.

However, the child may choose to remain out later to spend time with friends. In this situation, the parent may attempt to reach a compromise with the child by explaining their concerns for the child's well-being and the importance of

61

a good night's sleep. In addition, they could suggest a compromise, such as allowing the child to remain out later on weekends and holidays. Parent and child can prevent conflict and maintain a healthy relationship by communicating and finding a solution that works for both parties.

Another example of how to use negotiation and compromise to resolve a problem is making decisions regarding family responsibilities or duties. Children may feel overburdened or resentful if they are assigned an excessive number of duties or if they believe their responsibilities are unfair.

By negotiating with the child and finding ways to distribute tasks in a manner that is fair and doable for both parties, parents can help prevent conflicts and cultivate a greater sense of collaboration and teamwork within the family.

In another circumstance, discussions and compromises may be useful when selecting family activities or vacations. For instance, a parent may want to go on a nature hike with the family, while a child may prefer to visit a theme park. In this situation, the parent may attempt to negotiate with the child by highlighting the benefits of spending time in nature and the need for exercise. Alternately, they may recommend that the family indulge in both activities on separate days, or they may figure out a way to incorporate elements of both hobbies into a single outing.

Parent and child can benefit from shared experiences and strengthen their relationship by considering one another's preferences and coming up with a solution that works for all parties.

In addition to using negotiation and compromise to resolve individual conflicts, parents should set a positive example for their children by employing these methods. By demonstrating how to discuss and resolve problems calmly and politely, parents can help their children develop the skills necessary for successfully managing conflicts as they mature.

Building a strong and compassionate relationship with your child requires the ability to negotiate and compromise during conflicts. You can help your child develop the problem-solving skills necessary to manage conflicts successfully throughout their lives by attentively listening to your child's perspective, demonstrating a willingness to compromise, and modeling these skills for your child.

Chapter 10: Why is Corporate Communications So Important?

Corporate Communication is crucial for the health, recall, and expansion of any Brand or Organization. Here are some of the reasons why.

Brand Worth, Recall, and Recognition:

A brand's expansion is no longer dependent on advertising alone. The advertising industry is declining because the current generation prefers to make informed purchasing decisions and dislikes being sold to.

It is essential to develop audience-educational content, preferably through employee advocacy. Recently, this has become the most effective method for increasing Brand awareness and recall.

If all or many of your employees share Brand-related articles, content, or information on their personal social media accounts. As a result of each employee's large number of followers, the organization's and brand's reach is almost immediately expanded.

Individual / employee messages have significant value today. This ultimately results in increased brand recognition, recall, and revenue generation for the Brands and their respective Organizations.

Therefore, this format of CC strategy has a distinct yet indirect effect on the Organization's bottom line.

Employee Advocacy and Participation:

Employee Advocacy and Engagement Increases Productivity, Attracts Top Talent, and Aids in Retention.

Employee Engagement (EE) is a proven necessity for the achievement of all Organizational objectives.

An engaged worker will perform better and remain with the Organization for longer. In addition, they will serve as an example for other employees and new hires.

The Internal Communication component of an effective CC Strategy plays a crucial role in sustaining employee engagement.

When a CC strategy connects daily tasks to the organization's vision, mission, and objectives, everyone benefits.

A CC strategy should promote communication and allow employees to express their opinions, concerns, and ideas. This will enhance a culture of collaboration, creativity, and efficiency. When employees feel acknowledged and appreciated, they remain loyal to the organization.

Employees are the most effective spokespersons for the Organization. They are your greatest asset. Engaged personnel contribute to the success of the business.

Platforms for employee communications should serve as Knowledge Management portals that foster innovation in the workplace.

Employees should be encouraged to share industry and competitor updates via internal communication tools. In addition, communicating customer challenges, case studies, and successes with teams and senior management should be encouraged.

Knowledge Management Portals will aid in the development of new ideas and initiatives. Profitable ideas require departmental and management collaboration.

A good communications platform for employees eliminates the problem of squandering time searching for pertinent information and boosts productivity.

Effective internal communication fosters a knowledge-based and collaborative culture.

Companies are only as successful as their employees. The procedure of attracting talent is time-consuming and costly. A competent and efficient CC strategy can aid in attracting quicker and more cost-efficient talent.

Effective employee engagement results in increased referrals and is one of the most efficient and cost-effective hiring strategies.

A well-implemented employee advocacy program in Internal Communication transforms employees into Brand Ambassadors who promote open and essential positions on their social networks. Through corporate communication on social media, enormous savings on job advertisements and consultant fees are possible. Which will eventually impact the Organization's bottom line.

According to the guidelines provided by Corporate Communication, employees may use social media to exhibit the organization's culture. Examples include team-building activities, celebrations, progressive policies, corporate social responsibility, and other initiatives.

It provides excellent credibility for attracting talent and demonstrates that the organization has an exceptional work culture.

Chapter 11: Some Things Commonly Discovered In Conversations

Which sinister secrets do they share?

Edward Bennett Williams, Bill Clinton, and Frank Sinatra have much to teach us.

Successful communicators constitute the preponderance of successful members of society. The opposite is also largely accurate, which is not surprising. If you strive to improve your speaking skills, you will be successful. If you currently lack social status, you can improve your public speaking abilities to transform your social standing.

I am convinced that no successful person is bereft of self-expression. Even though they may not be excellent at public speaking or speaking in general, they must possess a certain level of speech in order to hold important positions.

Harry Truman is not considered an exceptional orator. However, many individuals laud him as an outstanding leader. Truman is particularly skilled at debating politics. He was an accomplished negotiator who spoke with self-assurance. He prefers to speak in simple, comprehensible terms as opposed to using flowery language. Truman's statement "The money stops here" (*), what a great orator he was, encapsulates the responsibilities of a president better than anyone else ever has.

Martin Luther King Jr. He is a highly knowledgeable speaker who consistently captivates the entire attention of his audience as if by magic. He has the ability to captivate an audience with only a modest microphone.

There will be further discussion of public speaking in a later chapter. I've had the opportunity to converse with numerous exceptional speakers, and I've concluded the following about their shared secrets:

GENERAL ADVICE

• They always approach situations from a novel perspective; • Their field of vision is expansive. • They are extremely inquisitive and always want to know more than you tell them. • They demonstrate a great deal of warmth and enthusiasm for what you are discussing. • They rarely discuss themselves.

• They can empathize and share; they can put themselves in your position to better understand what you're saying.

They are entertaining and have no problem making quips about themselves. Speakers who are the most acerbic about themselves are frequently the best speakers. • They have a distinct manner of speaking.

VIEW THINGS FROM NEW PERSPECTIVES

Successful communicators utilize this first secret frequently. An illustration is the late singer Frank Sinatra. If you have the good fortune to speak with Frank about music, you will soon become enamored because he is insatiably curious about everything. Frank has never boasted about his musical prowess; instead, he has extensive industry experience. In addition, Frank consistently offers novel observations and perspectives.

One evening in California, I was seated next to Frank at a gathering. He was requested to perform the well-known song "Remember?" by Irving Berlin. During my adolescence, this song was extremely popular. This melody is well-known and cherished by both young and old individuals. A heartfelt love ballad with a seductive melody for sensitive souls.

However, Frank's assertion that "I used to sing this song frequently" surprised me. Every time I perform, I sing a ballad. However, I will present in a distinct manner tonight. Comprehend why? because this music is so pitiful...

I murmured the lyrics briefly:

How about the evening? The night you professed your affection. Remember? Remember your vow. Remember by every star in the sky? (Do you recall that evening? The night you professed your affection. Do you recall, child? Be mindful of your pledges. The evidence for the oath is the constellations. Do you recall?").

"The individual in the post seems angry," Frank observed. I want to sing with greater passion this time. Frank also did. This demonstrates that he not only performs well, but also understands the meaning of the song.

Sinatra brought a new perspective to an ancient piece of text. I genuinely enjoy conversing with such individuals. He revitalized the gathering. Since then, whenever I hear the song "Remember," I endeavor to evoke new positive qualities or feelings. This is something I learned from Sinatra.

OPEN YOUR EYES,

New York City's mayor, Mario Cuomo, is a competent communicator. Andrew Cuomo's career in the entertainment industry is lucrative.

Andrew was a secretary working on urban housing development for the Clinton administration at the age of 30. Additionally, he engages in social activities. Andrew is a very intriguing individual with a versatile and complete personality. Having had multiple interactions with Andrew in Washington, I once told the mayor over the phone how much I valued our phone conversations. I believe he is virtually the optimal human being. It was explained to me by my father.

Andrew has had a close relationship with his elders ever since he was a young child. His grandparents are both grandparents. He was a constant source of questions and rapt attention. Mr. and

Mrs. Andrews were born in Italy in the early 20th century, when carriages were the primary mode of conveyance. There was no electricity, radio, or television at the time; only incurable diseases. At that time, individuals only attended a few lower grades of school, and word of mouth was the primary means of communication. As a consequence, Andrew received a wealth of information from his grandparents. He is adept at having a more profound and insightful perspective on society. Andrew has engaged in considerable amounts of listening and learning. Andrew has become increasingly attractive as a result of his insatiable inquiry and attentiveness.

Mayor Cuomo's emphasis prompted me to reflect. A proverb states, "A good day to learn a clever sieve." However, if you are motivated to study and attend to others, you can acquire a great deal of knowledge close to home. Everyone has both parents and grandparents. If you don't get a chance to converse with them, find other seniors with whom you can converse. By the time they are 80, 90, or even 100 years old, people have amassed a wealth of experience. By assimilating their life lessons and living capital, we can gain a deeper comprehension of our own existence.

When my father died, my mother labored to provide for us financially and nutritionally. She had to hire an elderly nanny to care for my siblings and clean the small Bensonhurst Street apartment because she was too occupied working at the factory (Brooklyn) to do so herself. The father of the 80-year-old woman fought in the North-South Civil War. As a young child, she met President Abraham Lincoln for the first time. And we had a pleasant discussion. Due to this, my childhood in Brooklyn provided me with a small window through which to view a component of American history. Similarly, you can gain a great deal from your time spent with adult family members. Share your thoughts on every topic with them and heed their advice. Someone with more life experience than you will unquestionably have a more developed perspective and be eager to help you broaden your horizons.

Those who are insatiably inquisitive about new topics are typically the most talkative. Because of this, they are paying close attention to you. And this is why they have a solid intellectual foundation.

Chapter 12: Developing the Relationships You Truly Desire

As we've seen, communication is neither naturally simple nor something that just occurs. The majority of us fail at relationships due to the common obstacles that make communication at times feel like an obstacle course. To communicate effectively, we must first identify the obstacles. However, the issue with impediments is that we frequently fail to recognize them. Because we've normalized them, they can appear to be facts.

Obstacles prevent us from being open to the communication process with another person. They create "mixed messages" concerning the information we are attempting to convey. When we have contradictory thoughts or emotions regarding the same subject, we are sending mixed messages. For instance, if you criticize a friend for not remaining in rehab, but you dropped out of college as a sophomore, you may be sending a mixed message. Although these are not identical, the other party may perceive the situation as "the pot calling the kettle black." This does not imply that the other person is correct or that the two events are comparable; however, this is how some individuals believe. It is a fortunate thing that we will not all have identical thoughts and experiences. The problem is that many individuals see differences as a source of division. But diversity of thought, people, and experiences fosters a relationship-rich environment. Unfortunately, we can lose out on relationship opportunities because we frequently focus on the obstacles rather than the person and the current situation.

Internal and external impediments exist for all of us. Internal impediments have to do with how our perceptions and experiences influence our relationship functioning and our relationship expectations. External obstacles are external influences that we cannot always control; however, they have a significant impact on how we operate in a relationship and can even alter our interactions with another person. I have identified seven communication barriers in total. First, we will analyze the four internal roadblocks in greater detail, followed by an analysis of the three external roadblocks' significance to the communication process.

The Four Internal Impasses

1. Honesty

You may be pondering how integrity can be an obstacle. It should, if anything, encourage communication. Interestingly, in enticing circumstances, honesty might necessitate deliberation. Sincerity can be subjective as well. How could this be? Ultimately, honesty appears to be straightforward; either a person is honest or they are not. Either what a person says is true or it is false. Unfortunately, there are numerous definitions of honesty. Consider the matter carefully. What are lies? What is an innocent lie? Exists a distinction between the two? What about leaving out certain details? Is this a lie? Is it possible to tell half-truths? What about being truthful, but not completely truthful? How does deception come into the picture? Clearly, "gray areas" of honesty are a reality. The majority of us do not consider nuances and specifics until we perceive someone to be operating in a gray area.

Consider, for instance, honesty in the context of infidelity. The wife inquires, "Where were you last night?" I was concerned when I did not hear from you prior to going to bed. What were you doing so late at night? The husband responds, "As you know, I was out with Eric and those individuals. Then Michael arrived to meet us, accompanied by his friends. You already know the outcome." Now, this may appear to be an extremely reasonable response. It makes logic. However, when listing all the guests, the spouse neglected to mention that Tiffany was also present. Tiffany is the housekeeper. Did he outright deceive his wife? Did he omit certain facts? Depending on your personal experiences and perspective, perhaps... or perhaps not.

Consider the most recent instance you either lied or felt you were lied to. How precisely did it become a lie? Did the other person believe it to be a lie? Similar to communication, there is a continuum of honesty. Sometimes you can ascertain the degree of honesty based on the source, despite your denial. For instance, are you more likely to trust information from your mother or your cousin? You may not be able to answer that question, as it may also hinge on the available data. If your acquaintance tells you that they struggle with infertility, you may be inclined to believe them, assuming that they have tried to conceive but have been unable to due to a medical condition. However, if your mother tells you that your cousin is struggling with infertility, you may be tempted to disbelieve her in the hopes that you will inquire with your cousin and report back to her. See how "honesty" can be used differently by different people and for various purposes?

Due to the gray area in which honesty can exist, we must recognize that the degree of honesty we have with ourselves is the most crucial. Consequently, we must communicate this honesty regarding the forbidden subject.

Regarding your relationships and the unaddressed forbidden topics, consider whether you have been completely truthful about your feelings, position, and attitude in the situation, as well as how you perceive the other person. Have you been completely truthful with the other individual? Reflect on whether you have conveyed your perceptions of the person's actions, words, and behaviors in the situation. The greatest strength you possess is your candor with another person about how these truths have affected you and the relationship as a result. Equally essential is being truthful about how your response in a given circumstance is directly related to these truths.

Chapter 13: Love and immunity: tested techniques for a healthier relationship

Enhanse your communication

Explain what is bothering you in a non-accusatory manner if you and your partner have a disagreement. Use all the caution you can muster to avoid saying, "You never" or "You always."

But for me, discretion is acceptable. Everything in your mind is unnecessary to state. I know you think you're going to erupt, but ask yourself if what you're about to say will help or harm your relationship.

Adopt a mindset of gratitude. Resentments demonstrate that gratitude benefits both the giver and the recipient. When one of you does something pleasant for the other – lets you peek in, holds the door when it's your turn – take a moment to express gratitude. Even if you're just expressing gratitude for small gifts, it can go a long way toward strengthening your relationship.

Use "hot words" when situations become contentious. Never respond when you are angry; if you need to calm down, leave the room or the house. Establish a "hot word" that each individual can use to signal to the other side, "I'm angry and we need to resume talking." "sansel" and "break" are examples of trendy words. Once both of you have calmed down, continue the conversation. The most effective way to fully comprehend what your spouse is saying is to ask clarifying questions. A clarifying question always begins with "What I understand you to be saying is... Is that correct?" This will give your partner the opportunity to concur or clarify what they meant. The objective is to always communicate with a level head.

Specify your need or desire in detail. You did not marry uour clone. Be cautious when communicating with your circle. Do not assume that he or she has read your mind or intuited your desires.

Display how much you adore your partner.

Write a love letter - the slas way to express oneself, which has been gradually superseded in modern society. In an era of virtual communication, couples may benefit from exchanging and/or receiving a handwritten note – not an email, not a text message, but something more personal.

Take a sla collectively. Courle who are not engaged in any joint activities are living "parallel lives" like children in parallel play; there is no genuine connection. connection. Without shared time and activities, ntmasu is harmed. The benefits are numerous. Learning together alleviates monotony, routine, and tedium and enables us to view our lives in a new light. This keeps the creative juices flowing, which makes a story more engaging. It also affords the opportunity for new and intriguing sonveration, either during the astvtu or afterward. The act of preparing a meal and sharing it with your spouse creates a sense of safety and security in your relationship.

Go beuond plain "I love uou" remarks. Utilize expressive language. When sourle au specifically, "I love how enthuats (or sourageou, or sarng, or thoughtful...) you are," t reaches the heart. It's like providing gold if you include details about the asteroids that were seized.

Even inexpensive fast-food dates are essential. You don't have to spend a fortune in order to spend time with your significant other; plan a weekly date night. As a street evangelist, we have a monthly budget of $100. Once per month, we dine at a Japanese restaurant. The remaining three weeks, we visited Chsk-Fl-A or Subwau. We simply take a detour to have some alone time. It is always extremely invigorating."

However, you can have a date night at home, even with your child. Manu sourle are assaulted at the end of the day, and dinner is flung onto the table. Make the dinner table more intimate by using dishware that matches, a vase of flowers, and dimmer lighting. Even with children, who frequently learn from what they oberve their parents do rather than what their parents au, these specific actions endear the couple and elicit speculation.

Create a memento that commemorates a special moment you and your partner shared. Find a favorite photograph of the two of you and have it printed on a refrigerator magnet or a large photo frame. I did this roughly seven years ago with a beach photo we took one summer. At the losal office supply store, I discovered a box of rrntable magnets. I created a large refrigerator magnet with our photograph using our home computer and printer, and it is still on our refrigerator to this day.

Reference to the quoted individual does not constitute an endorsement of the individual's external work or of their respective organizations.

4.2 Be Directly to the Point

Occasionally, speakers use less effort and fewer words to get their point across. So, keep your sentences brief and pleasant. Avoid appearing excessively regretful or over-explaining your reasons for declining.

You can also demonstrate assertiveness through nonverbal communication. Maintain eye contact with the person with whom you are conversing, face them directly, and speak firmly enough for all of them to hear you. While assertiveness requires expressing one's opinion, comprehension is also essential. Permit us to respond to your comments as well. The concept is to be amenable to imposing one's beliefs on others. Listening may make it easier for you to approach the topic at hand; knowing that you will grant the other person the floor will make you feel less aggressive and guilty for being forthright.

Nevertheless, assertiveness can be more challenging depending on the topic. It is one thing to tell your friend the truth about her new haircut, but quite another to confront a colleague about their habit of taking credit for your work. Recognize that it will initially be uncomfortable.

It may be preferable to begin a disagreeable conversation with a disclaimer. This is particularly helpful if the recipient is unfamiliar with your direct address. Start the conversation by informing the other party that you need to discuss a sensitive topic with them. You want them to be truthful because you do not want to generate resentment or difficult situations in whatever situation you are in, be it a class presentation, a relationship discussion, or a workplace argument. If you disagree with a family member or close acquaintance, tell them that you value your relationship with them enough to be honest.

Moreover, if you are reticent to be direct due to anxiety, remember that most people appreciate it. After all, directness and honesty are frequently used interchangeably. It is an act of kindness and courtesy that encourages others to do the same. The more you establish yourself and practice communication, the more others will respect you, even if they disagree with you. As unpleasant as it may be for your subject to embrace the truth, it is often the best course of action to be honest with them. Just do not behave in an annoying manner.

Chapter 14: In the digital age, persuasive communication

In our fast-paced, always-connected society, it is easy to overlook the importance of face-to-face communication. As anyone who has ever had a heart-to-heart conversation knows, however, there is something special about being able to look another person in the eye and share your thoughts and emotions. When executed effectively, writing can be an immensely potent means of connecting with others. However, the majority of us do not compose eloquent messages or emails, and this hurried substitute for meaningful connection can be challenging.

Texting

It is now one of the most prevalent forms of communication. This form of communication can easily lead to misunderstandings and conflict, despite the fact that texts are a convenient way to remain in touch with friends and family. To ensure that your texts convey the intended message, it is essential to consider both the content and the tone. The following are some effective messaging guidelines:

Be straightforward and concise regarding the text's subject matter. The recipient should be able to comprehend your message without having to speculate or interpret it. Avoid using abbreviations and vernacular with unfamiliar individuals.

It is also essential to consider the tone of your text. Often, emoticons and expressive language are more effective than actual words at conveying the intended tone. Using more emojis and exclamation points in your text, for instance, can help you come across as playful or welcoming. A well-placed emoji or humorous GIF can add personality and humor to your texts if you believe it's necessary.

Remember that texts are frequently read out of context, so it is essential to choose your words cautiously. If you are uncertain of how the recipient will interpret your writing, it is prudent to err on the side of caution. Be forthright. If it sounds too straightforward or clinical, add a gif or an emoji. Consider that the recipient may misunderstand what you've written, and be concise. Keeping these guidelines in mind, messaging can be an effective means of communication.

Chapter 15: The Most Effective Way To Communicate Within A Relationship

Correspondence in relationships can be the difference between significant areas of strength for an association and a conflict-filled relationship that ends in frustration. Improving one's communication skills is essential.

Commit TO Genuine Association

The most erroneous assumption about how to communicate in a relationship is that written communication is equivalent to verbal communication. At its core, correspondence in relationships is about collaborating and utilizing your verbal, written, and physical skills to meet your partner's needs. There is no need to concentrate on establishing casual conversation. It involves comprehending your partner's perspective, providing support, and letting them know you are their number one fan.

Especially in long-term relationships, it is simple for genuine connection and enthusiasm to diminish. However, the primary key to enhancing communication in a relationship is to acknowledge that you are no longer communicating as you once did. Communicate with your partner about reviving your relationship and provide a starting point. In the event that your partner isn't prepared, simply remain calm. Connections are not about receiving, but rather about giving. You can still order a significant number of these procedures without your partner's consent, and you may attempt to motivate them to respond.

2. Recognize YOUR Correspondence STYLES

Before attempting to determine how to further develop correspondence in a relationship, you should recognize that not everyone has the same correspondence manner. Latent, forceful, quiescent forceful, and emphatic are the four primary correspondence styles. Detached communicators keep their emotions to themselves, whereas Forceful communicators are direct and forceful, but have difficulty forming genuine relationships with others. Inactive forceful communicators avoid conflict and use ridicule to avoid genuine communication. The most effective correspondence is composed of individuals who are in touch with their emotions and have the ability to effectively convey them.

Also included in correspondence styles are our metaprograms, or the manner in which we respond to data. Some individuals prefer verbal communication, others prefer physical contact, while others are more visual or prefer gift-giving over verbal expressions of emotion. You likely know which correspondence style you prefer, but what can you say about your partner?

Correspondence and connections are unique. Recognizing this will facilitate a healthy relationship with your partner. Your partner may be telling you precisely what they want, but you must be mindful of how they communicate this information. If there is a misunderstanding, you will miss out on an incredible opportunity to build trust and intimacy, and you will both be disappointed.

Observe your partner's responses to a variety of insightful signals north of a short period of time as you work to improve your communication skills. Does the person appear to respond primarily to seeing and watching? Hearing and talking? Or conversely, contacting and acting? For instance, if your partner is more receptive to language, tone, and other audible cues, visually connecting and subtle glances may not be communicating as much as you believe. You are sending them messages, but they are not receiving them. Nonetheless, if you are a hearing person and your partner is a feeling person, keep in mind that "I love you" may not be sufficient. Develop your affection through physical contact, and do so frequently.

Significant avenues of affection are also crucial factors that make a relationship practically ideal.

Chapter 16: Developing Your Own Self-Confidence Step By Step

It could require time and effort to gain confidence. In addition, what benefits you now may not help you in the future. However, there are many things you can do to improve your self-confidence and perception of your abilities.

Kindness to Oneself

Recognize your unkind thoughts and resist them. To accomplish this, consider speaking to yourself as you would a close friend. How might others perceive this? Does anything indicate that this might not occur? You may be able to think more logically and methodically after answering these questions.

Remember that it is acceptable to make errors. When you make a mistake, you must assume full responsibility for it.

Do not evaluate yourself against others. Consider the fact that social media users meticulously select or filter the images they post. Moreover, they frequently fail to depict how people actually live.

Repeat uplifting affirmations to yourself. For example, you may say to yourself in the mirror every morning, "I am enough" or "I am worth it."

Look after Yourself

Try to get sufficient rest, consume a healthy diet, stay active, spend time in nature, and avoid using narcotics and alcohol.

Accentuate the Positive

You could recognize your accomplishments. Additionally, you may compile a list of your positive qualities for future reference. This could be applicable to any compliments you receive, even if you initially do not believe them. Over time, you might begin to develop a new perspective on yourself.

Spend Time with Individuals

Have joy with your loved ones, cultivate relationships with those you trust and identify with, and be kind to them. These individuals will embrace you precisely as you are.

Volunteering, lending a hand, or using your skills to aid a friend or family member can raise your self-esteem.

Do Activities You Enjoy

This may include swimming, playing video games, and listening to music. Even if only for a few minutes, allow yourself to enjoy yourself without feeling guilty.

Perform Confidence Even If You Don't Feel It

To develop a confident demeanor in front of others, you can begin by rehearsing conversation and posture in front of a mirror. However, if you can maintain it, you may realize after a while that you are no longer acting.

Try Something Different

By attempting something new, you may gain a new skill and meet new people. It may involve learning a few words of a foreign language, mastering a musical instrument, creating art through painting or drawing, or enrolling in a class or joining a sports team. You could do it for enjoyment, or you could set goals to track your progress.

Chapter 17: The Impact of Our Words on the World

Words carry weight. Their significance solidifies perspectives that shape our worldview, motivate our actions, and ultimately form our beliefs. Our visceral responses when we read, say, or hear them give them their power. Simply uttering the word "fire" while grilling, working, or in a crowded theater will evoke three distinct but equally potent emotional and energetic responses.

The Positive Lifestyle

According to quantum physics, physical matter does not exist, and everything is solely energy in various vibrational states. Nobel Prize-winning physicist Werner Heisenberg once stated, "Atoms or elementary particles themselves are not real; they form a world of potentialities or possibilities rather than one of things or facts." The inexhaustible variety of delicate frequencies at which this energy vibrates gives birth to all the diverse phenomena we observe in the universe. In recent years, the question of whether our universe is truly a holographic experience has been the subject of extensive research, and it appears that this is a very near approximation of reality.

Consequently, existence appears to be a flow of energy rather than a collection of material objects. This means that if we remain conscious of the energy we emanate and the emotions we experience, we can consciously alter our frequency and manifest the reality we desire. When we're feeling down about something, we can choose to alter our perspective. With a new perspective and a higher, more positive energetic vibration, we have a much greater chance of attracting good into our lives than when we repeat the same errors with resentment.

Although we are frequently unaware of the words we use, read, and are exposed to, words are immensely potent tools that can be used to increase our energy and improve our lives. Yes, even the comments of others have the ability to affect our vibration. Spending a few minutes with someone who constantly complains and uses foul language will deplete your energy. Words are extremely potent, so choose your companions (and words) with care.

Chapter 18: Obtain People's Support for Your Vision Before All Else

If you are in the sales industry, you are well aware that individuals do not purchase goods and services. They invest in the fantasy of possessing or utilizing the product or service. The same mentality should be employed when searching for individuals to assist you in running your business. Nobody will collaborate with you based on the product or service you provide, unless you are the next Elon Musk or Steve Jobs, of course. Instead, they will base their decision on the magnitude of your vision and whether it correlates with their values and life path.

Before discussing the mechanisms of selling your vision, however, it is important to distinguish between an idea and a vision. There are countless concepts circulating on social media, in business meetings, and pretty much everywhere else. Ideas are typically what inspire entrepreneurs to start businesses, but they will not aid them in sustaining their enterprises. This is because ideas can alter and change and do not require a concrete foundation.

Visions differentiate enterprises. They are the stabilizing force that defines the nature of the organization, its interests, and its goals. Visions persuade individuals, not ideas. What's the explanation? As a result of the opportunities they present. The reality is that we are all desperate to be a part of something greater than ourselves; to support a mission that challenges our minds, promotes personal development, and offers career advancement.

According to a survey conducted in South Korea, 70% of job seekers are keen to work for a startup company. They were permitted to cite any reason for their decision, and the most frequently cited reasons were the potential learning opportunities (35%), the appealing employee welfare programs (29.5%), and the propensity for startups to have a horizontal work culture (27.2%) (Hyeong-woo, 202). Such studies demonstrate the competitive advantage that entrepreneurs can have over more established businesses. By focusing on presenting a compelling vision, you can attract the skilled, motivated, and diligent individuals you seek.

There are three stages you can take to create, promote, and attract the appropriate individuals with your vision. These three stages consist of:

Step 1: Create the Objective

Okay, so you've been inspired to launch a business by a brilliant idea. First, you will need to formulate a clear vision for this grand concept. To accomplish this, you must concentrate on your "why." Consider the significance of this idea for some time. What issues does it intend to address? How will it unite individuals? Or how will it improve the lives of people?

If you want your "why" to have an impact, it must be greater than you. In other words, you will not establish a business solely for the purpose of making money. This is still insufficient to establish a sustainable business. Think greater. Much much larger. Your "why" should advance society, make a positive difference in people's lives, or address community-based challenges.

If you cannot articulate a compelling "why" for your current business notion, you should reconsider it. Pursuing a vision that does not address a problem or improve people's lives is not worth the effort. Return to the design board and consider additional potent ideas, then repeat step one.

Chapter 19: Identifying and regulating emotions

Emotions play a central role in communication and have a substantial influence on how we convey ourselves and interpret the words and actions of others.

In order to communicate effectively and develop healthy relationships, we must be aware of and in control of our emotions.

This chapter will examine the function of emotions in communication and how to effectively control and express them.

Body:

The function of feelings in communication:

Emotions can have a significant impact on both verbal and nonverbal communication.

For instance, anger or frustration can cause us to speak more openly or use more aggressive body language, whereas anxiety or fear can make us less likely to speak up or express ourselves.

In order to communicate effectively, it is essential to be aware of how our emotions influence our communication and to attempt to regulate them.

Methods for controlling and expressing emotions:

There are several techniques that can help us effectively manage and convey our emotions:

Pause for a moment and consider how you are feeling. Before responding, this can help you better understand and regulate your emotions.

Utilize "I" statements to communicate your emotions and demands. For instance, "When you interrupt me, it makes me feel as though my thoughts and feelings are not valued."

To calm your emotions, practice deep breathing or other relaxation techniques.

Obtain assistance from a trusted friend, therapist, or other confidant if you struggle to manage your emotions.

Chapter 20: Make The Effort To Communicate

They say that time is the best gift you can ever give someone because you are essentially giving them a piece of your existence that you can never get back. Since Quality Time is my primary mode of affection, I will generally concur. How would you set aside a few minutes for a relationship while being tugged in a hundred different directions?

One of the most common complaints among couples is that their partner does not exert sufficient effort or energy into the relationship, to the point where it has become completely imbalanced.

In daily life, we create opportunities for the things that have the greatest impact on us. To prioritize your relationship, you must begin setting aside time to concentrate on your partner.

Organize Routine Excursions

All of us are occupied with work, travel, and family responsibilities; if you are unable to consistently schedule a date with her, make up for it by transporting her away for a weekend getaway.

Occasionally, we as a whole experience chasms in our relationships. Things become monotonous and tiresome. Sounds normal? Make an attempt to escape your daily routine. Instead of frequenting the same establishments, you should visit the recently opened hotspot. Attend a springtime craftsmanship exhibition. Together, familiarize yourselves with another activity or expertise.

If being in love is important to you, you must make time for a romantic relationship. Assuming that you want to assign a few projects to ensure that you leave the office on time every Friday evening, then make it happen.

Purchasing season tickets to a venue is an effective method for encouraging more date nights. If it's now paid for and you realize there's an empty seat waiting for you, you must find a way to leave.

Moreover, if proximity is essential, write it down. It's not ideal to place it on the schedule, but if that's the only way to guarantee its success, write it in large letters and underline it in red.

Ignore Your Telephones.

Quality is the catchphrase for Value Time. It is difficult to connect with someone who is more focused on iTunes.

We're dependent on our devices enough.

From rest to intimacy, research demonstrates there are innumerable reasons why leaving your phone outside the bedroom at night is a good idea. You should also prohibit them from the dinner table and nighttime activities. In the early stages of a relationship, you may not be able to devote as much time and energy to your companion as you would like, so you must make the most of the time you have.

Reduce Time Spent on Correspondence

When circumstances permit, sleep concurrently and incorporate correspondence into your daily routine. Utilize the time spent preparing for bed and snuggling up at night to connect with others.

Even if you are in different regions of the world, take a few moments each night to check in with each other internally.

Facetime is a wonderful innovation, but calls are also acceptable.

Your partner is executing a task today; they have educated you previously. It is an agreement, a meeting, or a small assignment.

Recall through your recent conversations something that is occurring today, and send them a brief instant message or phone call regarding it.

"Trust that the medical examination was successful!" These snippets of association reinforce your sense of belonging to a group, that it's you and them against the world.

In long-distance relationships, partners develop a daily schedule of task division.

For instance, you typically empty the trash can while your partner shears the grass. You are responsible for cleansing the Dartington Precious stone, while your partner is responsible for the crystal fixtures.

For a five-minute love mission, assume one of your partner's typical positions and perform it for them. Try not to approach them a short time later like a giddy child requesting praise; instead, complete their request and wait for them to discover it.

Before the Internet, the world was divided into two types of people: those who could remember birthdays and anniversaries and those who lived in culpable hysteria. Fortunately, we can now all appear intelligent and considerate by setting up reminders for all the important dates in our and our partner's lives.

Sit down with the calendar application on your cell phone, computer, or tablet and input all the important dates: your wedding anniversary, your partner's birthday, the anniversary of your most memorable date... Make them an annual occurrence, and schedule a reminder seven days beforehand. Blast! No more hysteria.

Additionally, make it easy for your partner to pursue the things that bring them joy. If they appear exhausted and stressed, give them a shower and prepare dinner. To see a film that you recognize you will despise, you should buy tickets for themselves and a companion and drive them to the theater.

Assuming that observing Strictly motivates them, you should set up an automatic recording for the series. The happier your partner is, the happier your relationship will be.

www.ingramcontent.com/pod-product-compliance
Lightning Source LLC
Chambersburg PA
CBHW060512030426
42337CB00015B/1862